funnyPharm

Graham Harrop

ISBN: 1535130717
ISBN-13: 978-1535130174

FOR PHARMACISTS AND THEIR
ASSOCIATES EVERYWHERE

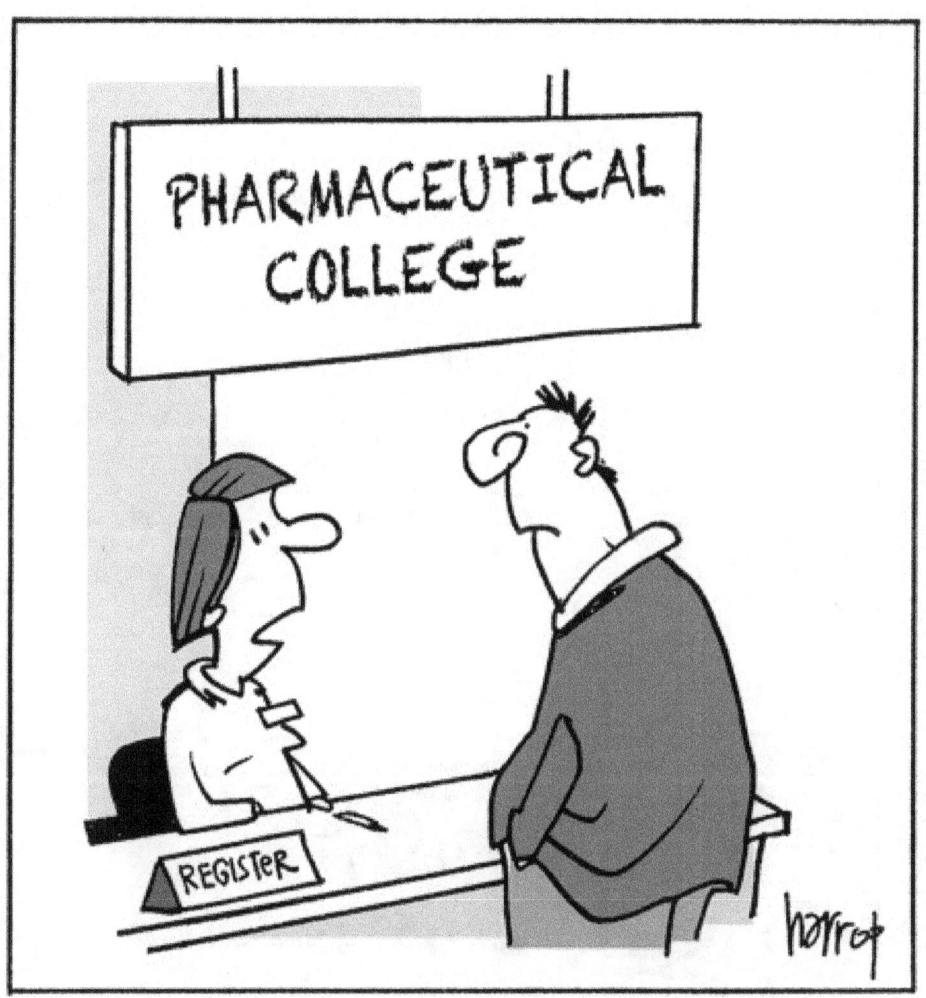

That's right - even if you already own a
white coat, we still expect you to take the course!

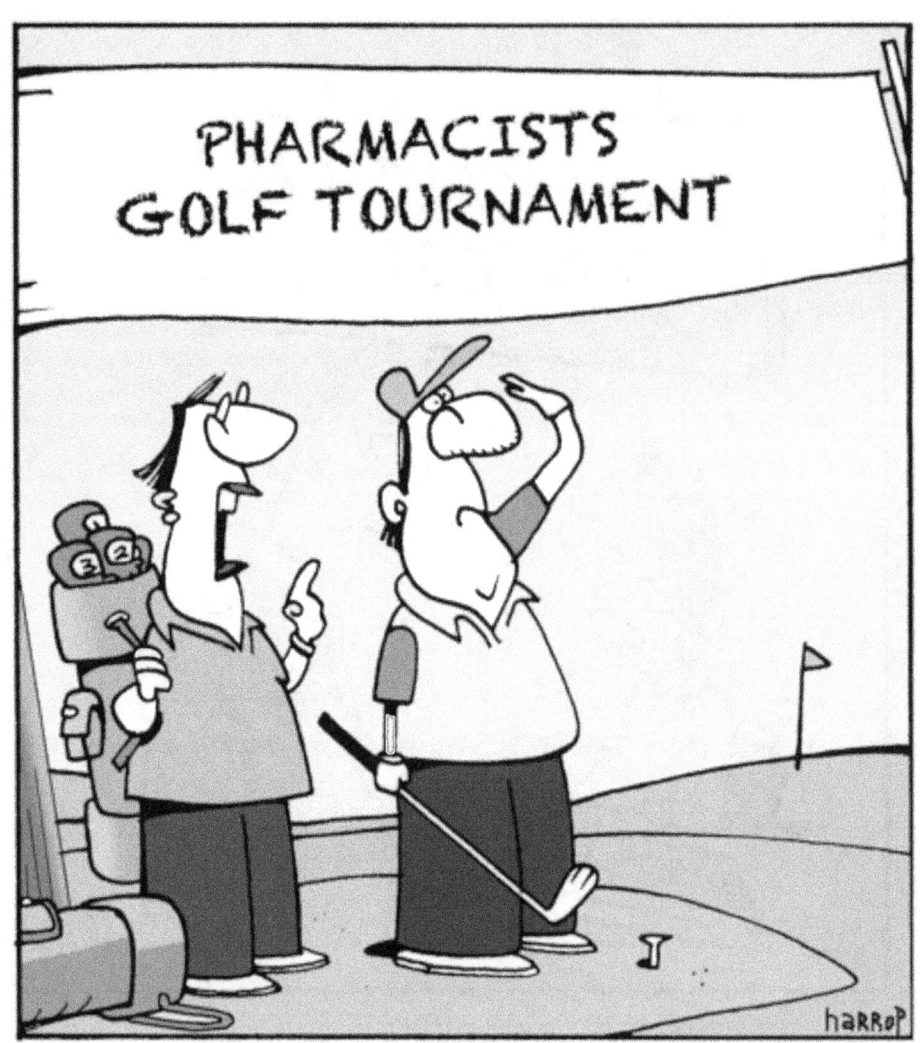

You've hit another pharmacist...
the good news is that he's wearing
a safety cap.

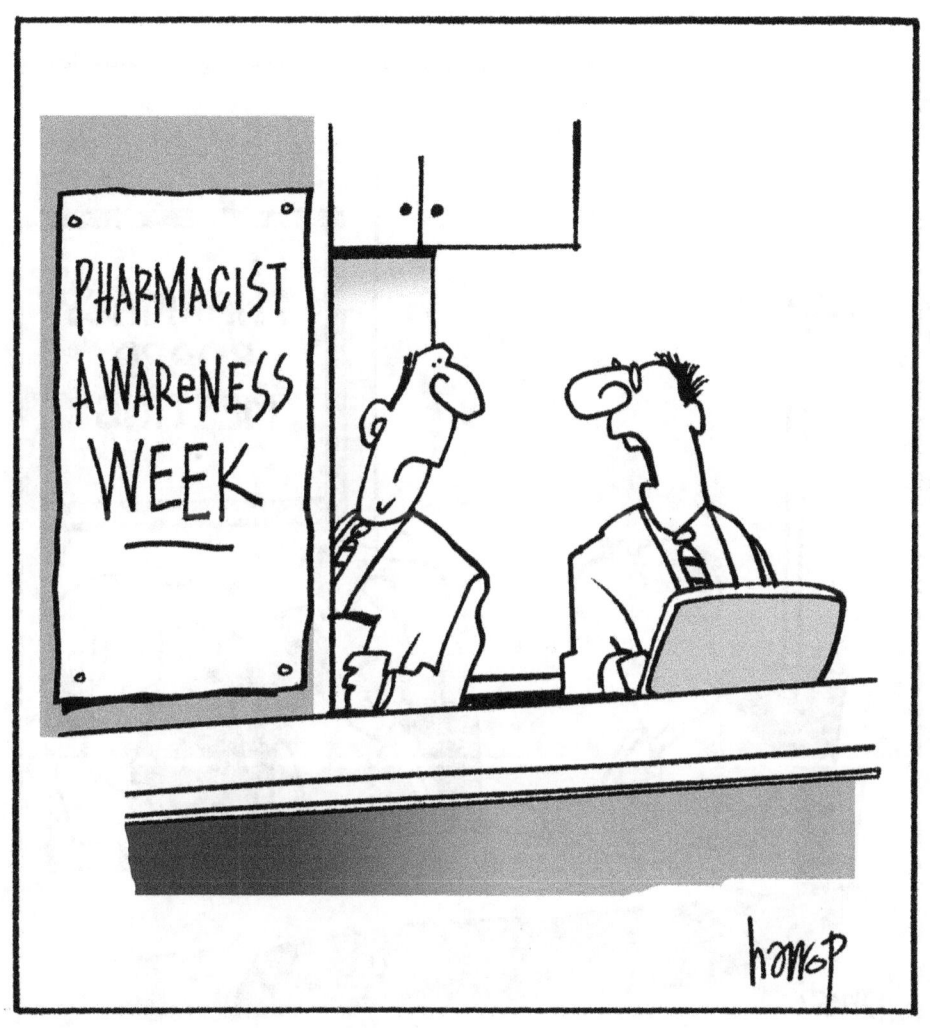

Of *COURSE* I'm aware of you, Waldren!
Now go back to work!

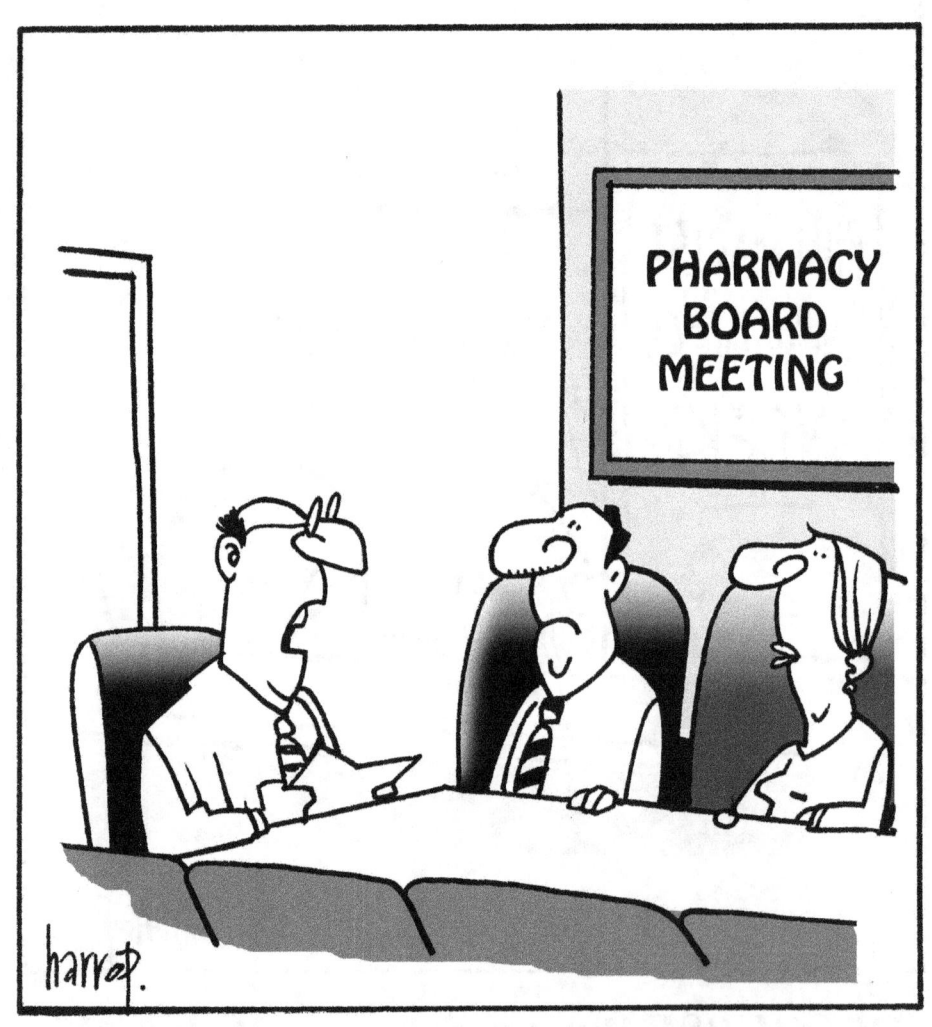

**I don't care if we *ARE* on Twitter ...
stop calling me 'dude' ... !**

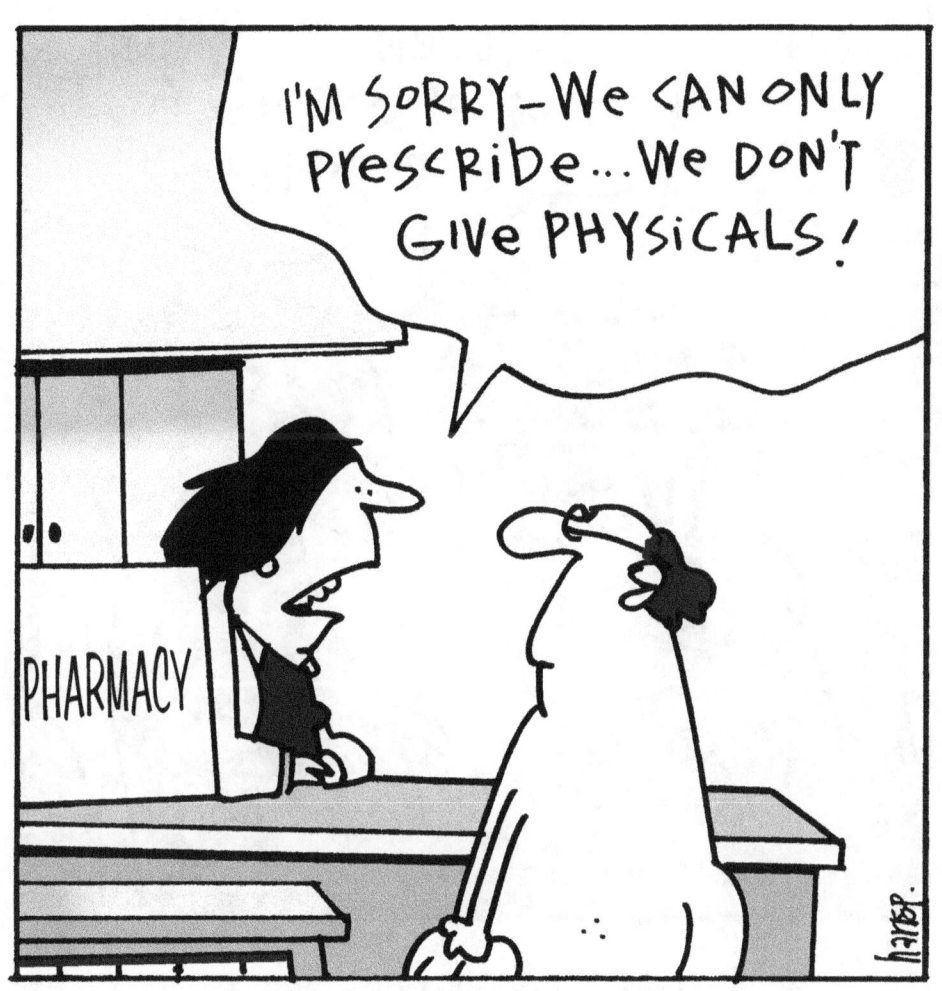

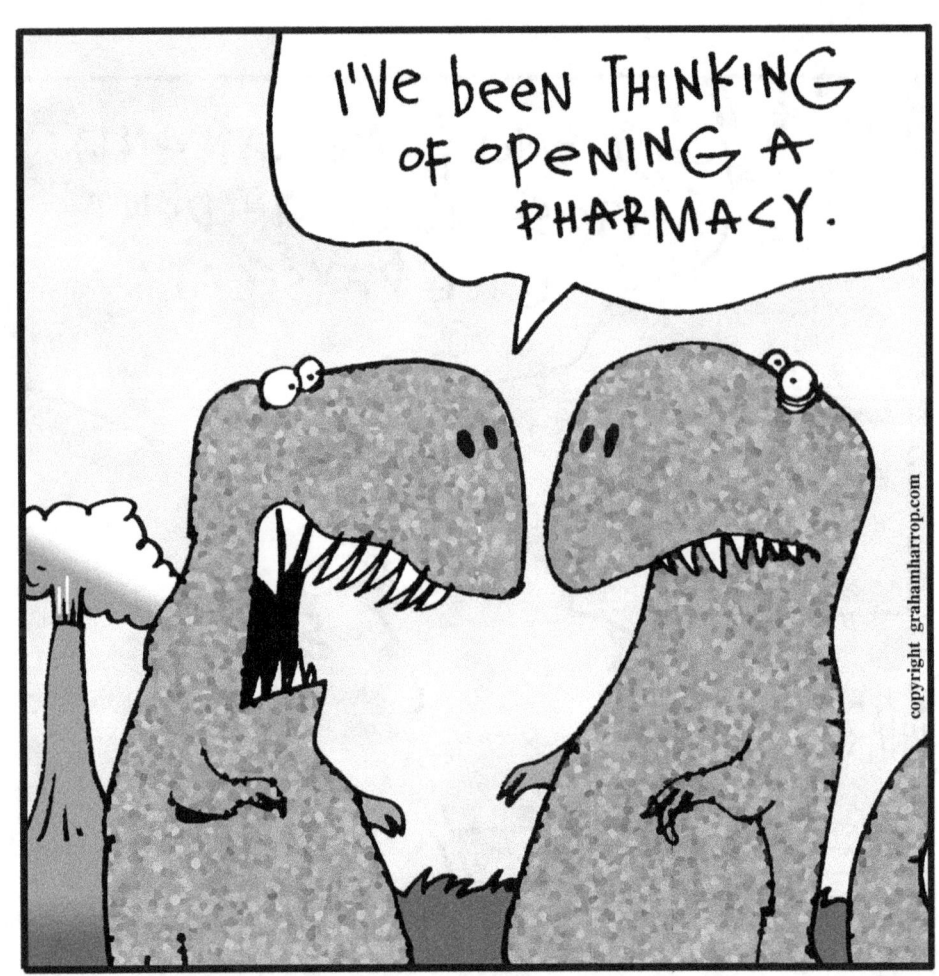

tyrannosaurus R~X~

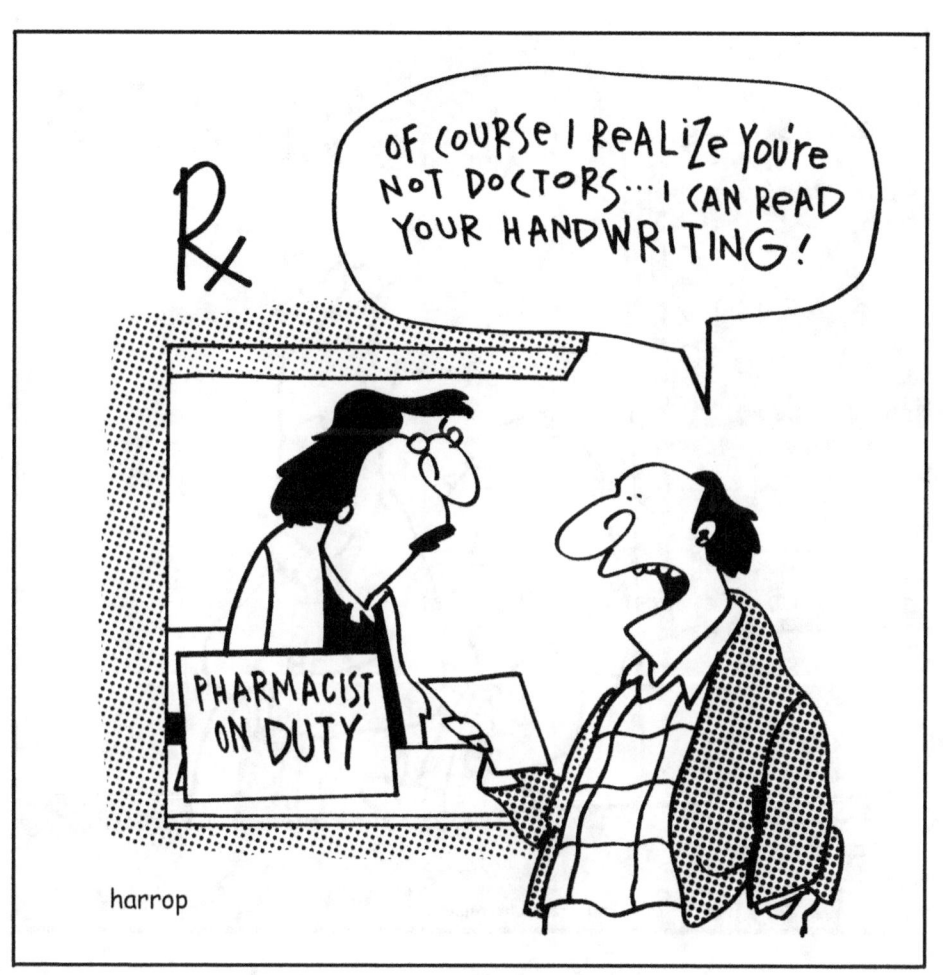

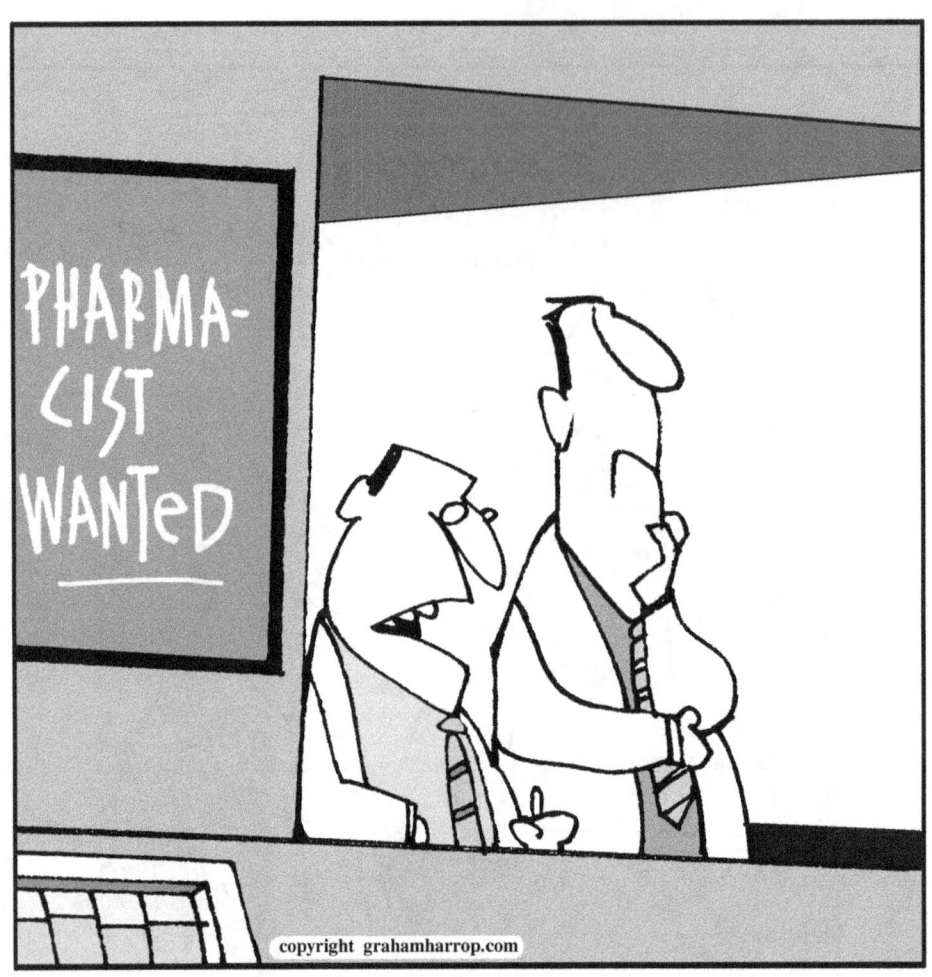

Maybe we should drop the 'leaps tall buildings in a single bound' requirement...

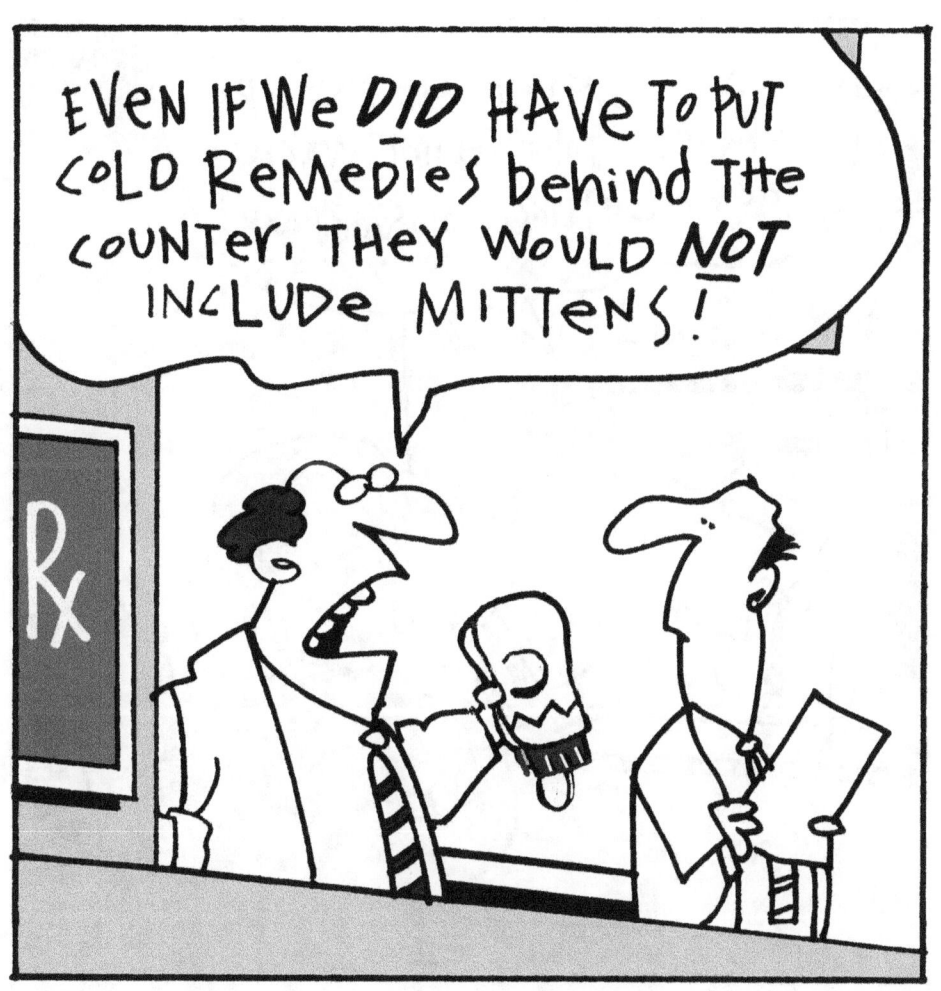

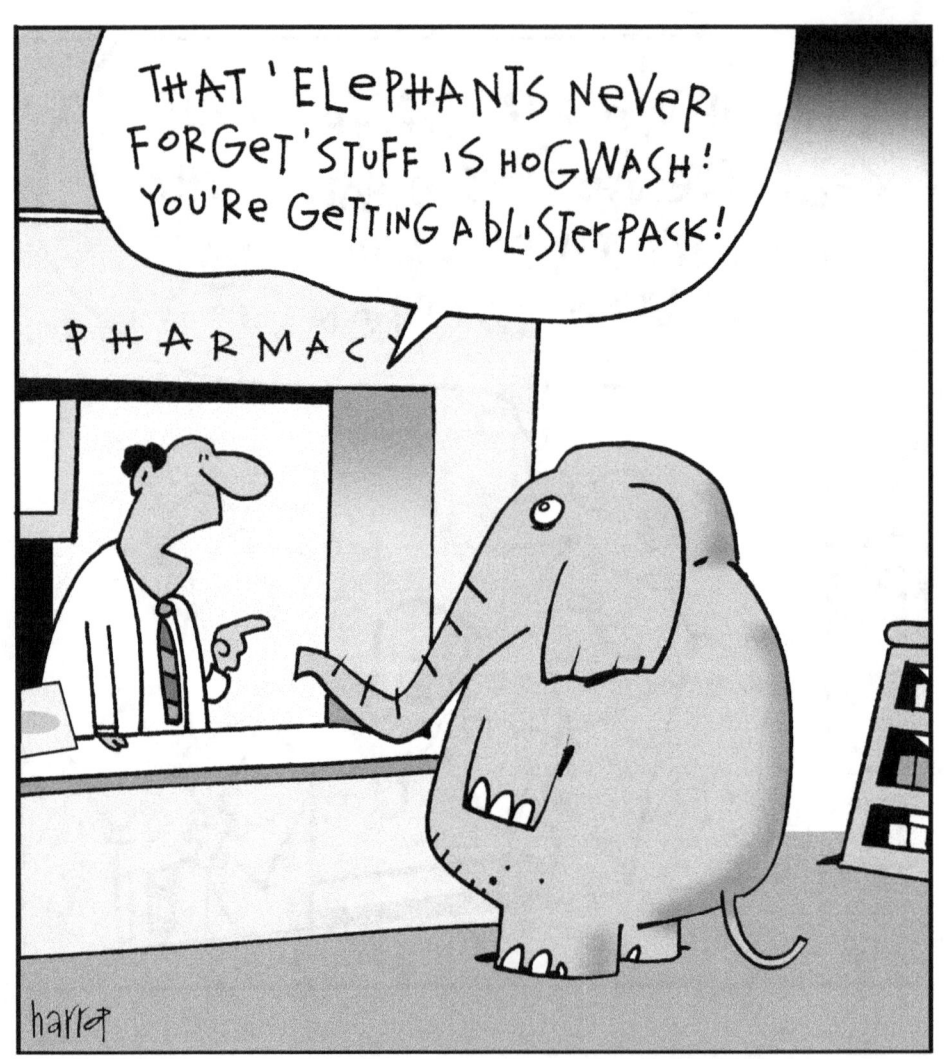

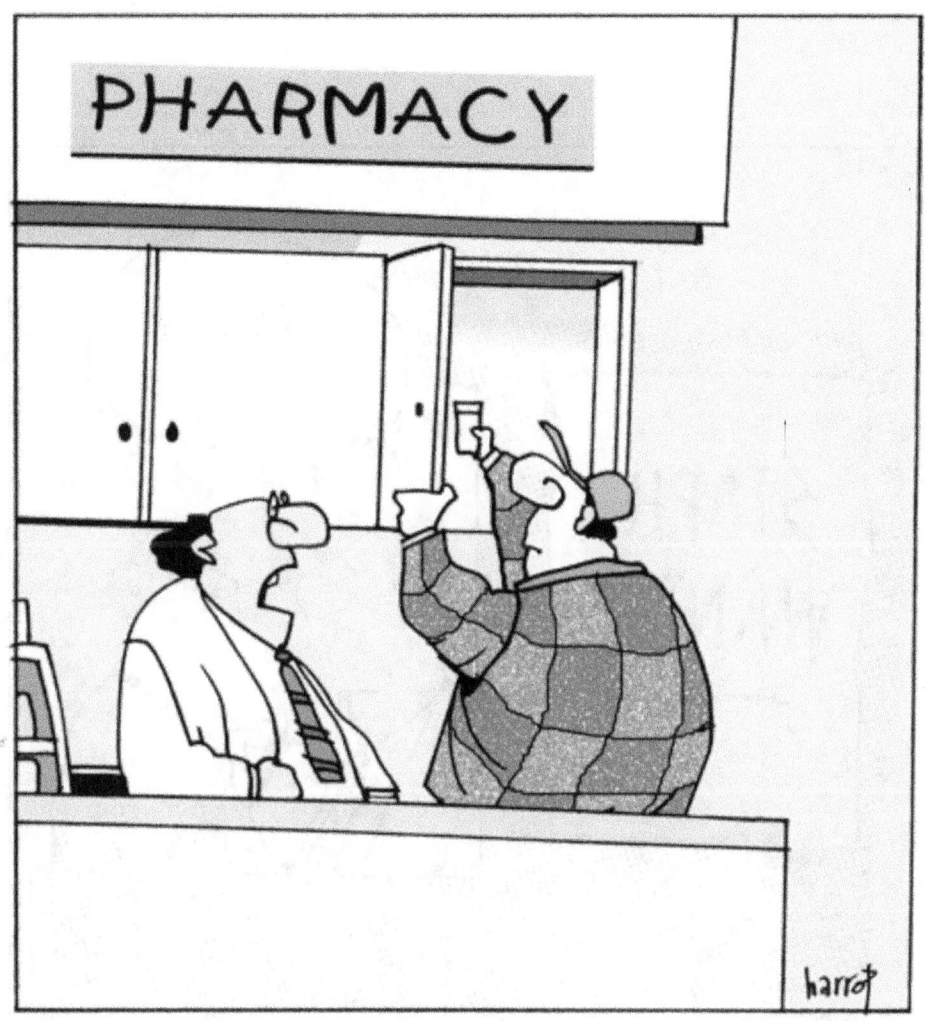

We're ALL in a hurry these days, Mr. Fossy, but if you don't mind - I'll dispense the medication!

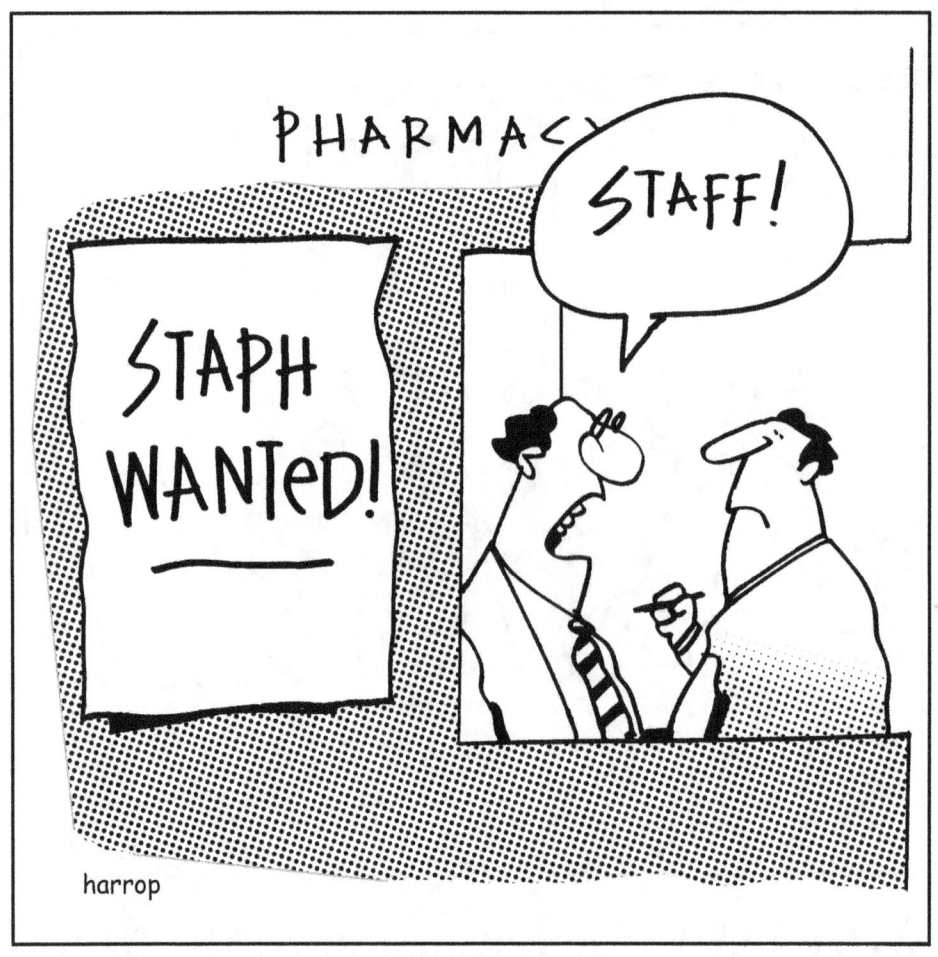

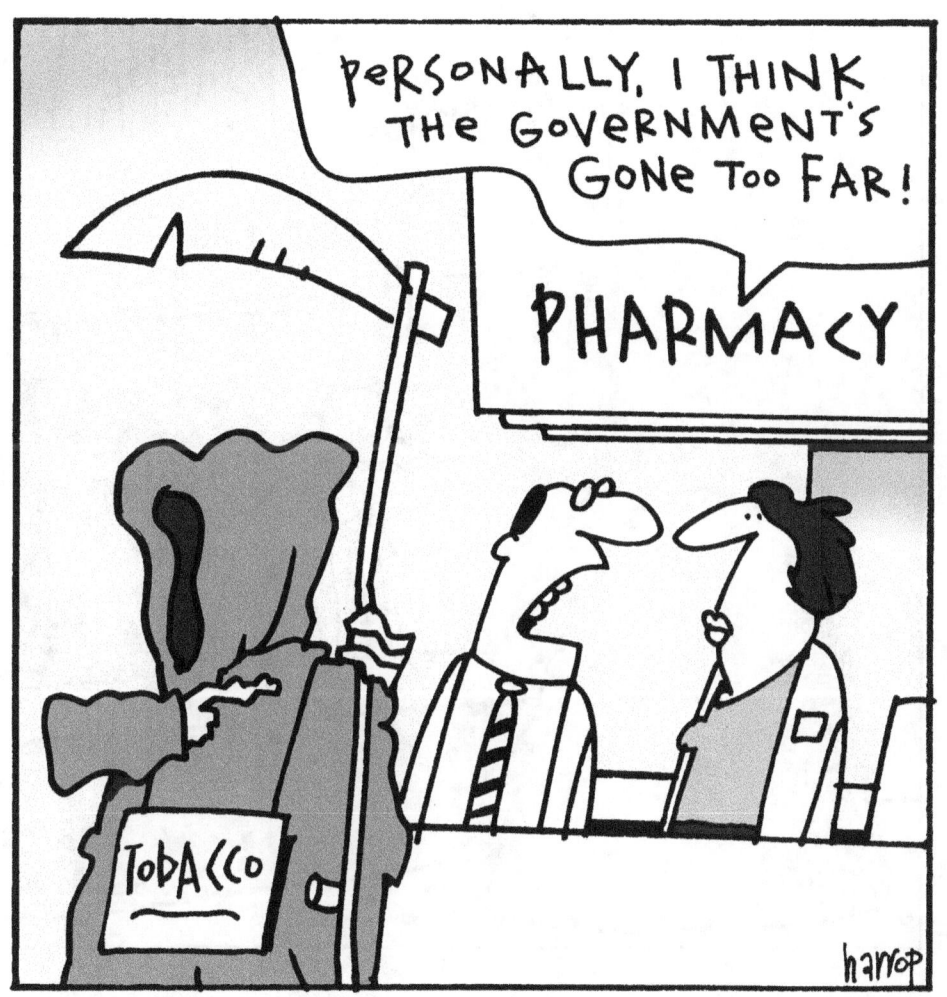

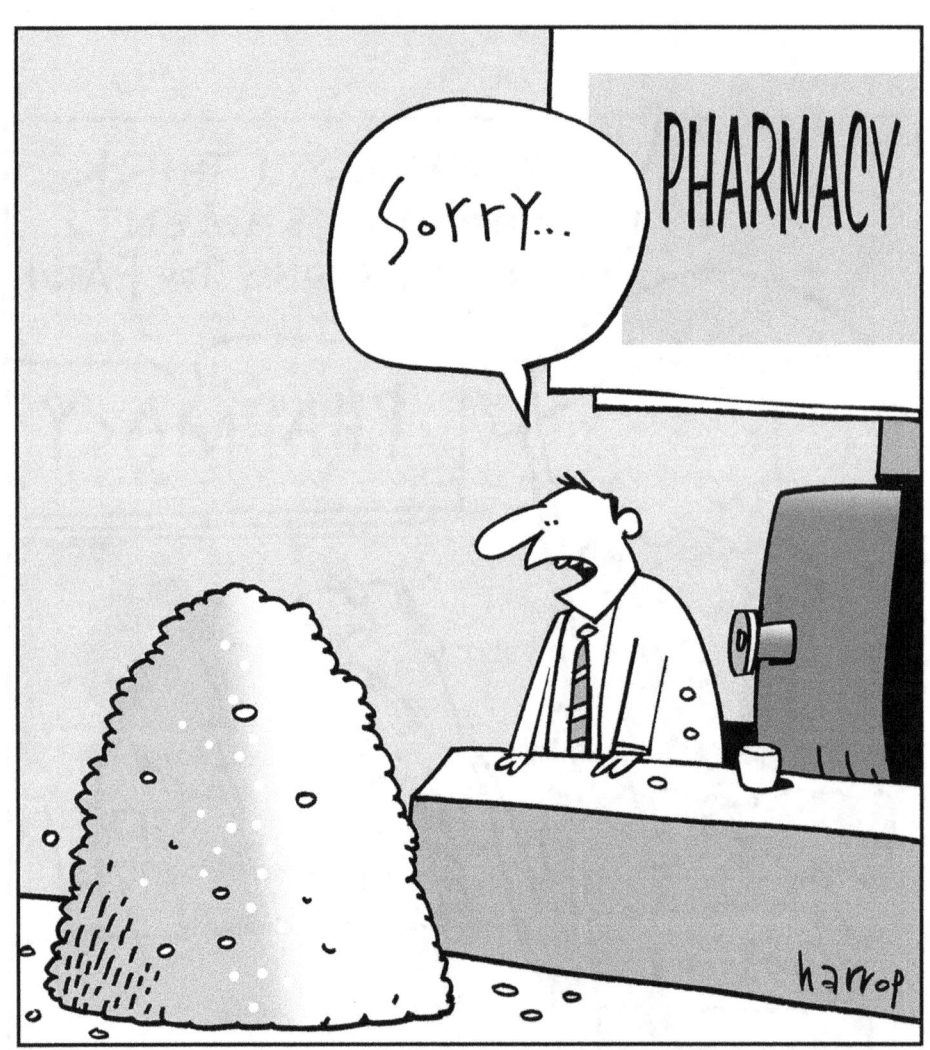

The first robotic pill dispensing machine
still had a few bugs to be worked out...

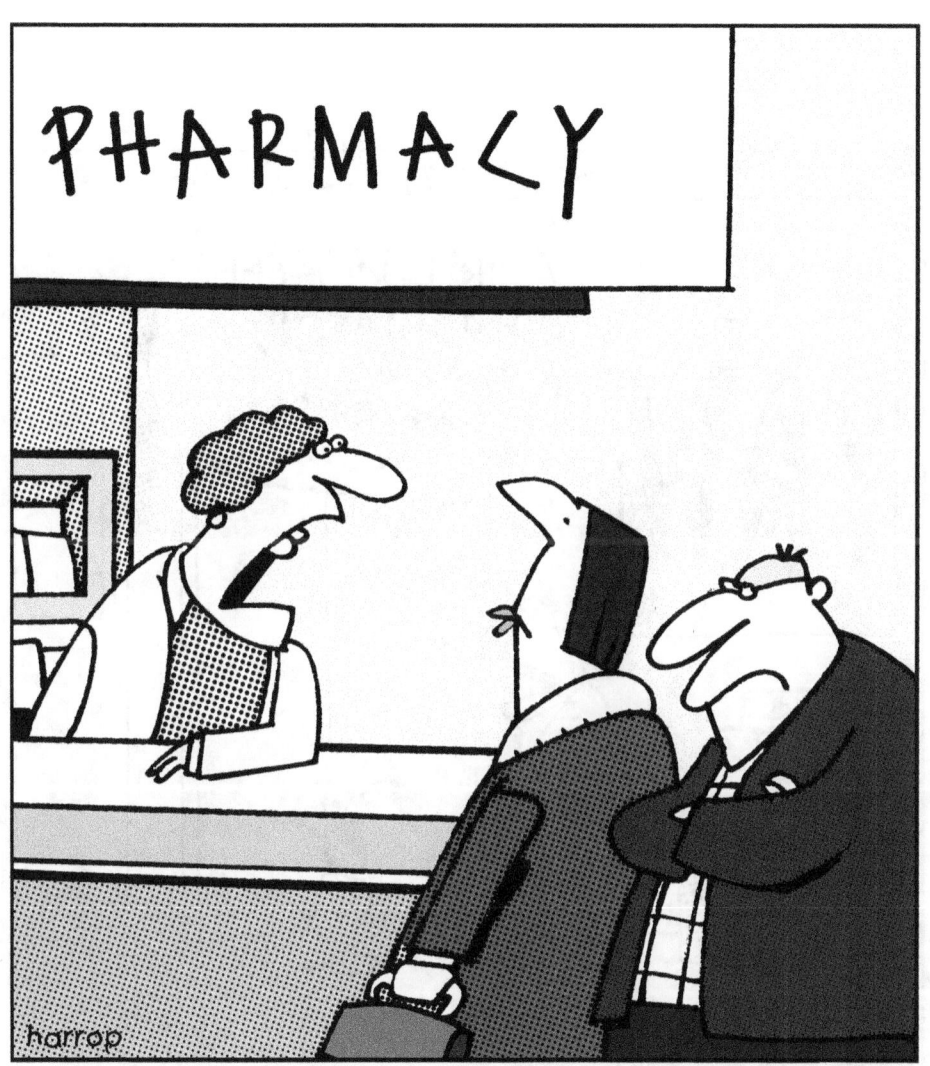

I'm sorry - but to prescribe something for a 'pain in the butt' - it has to be your own!

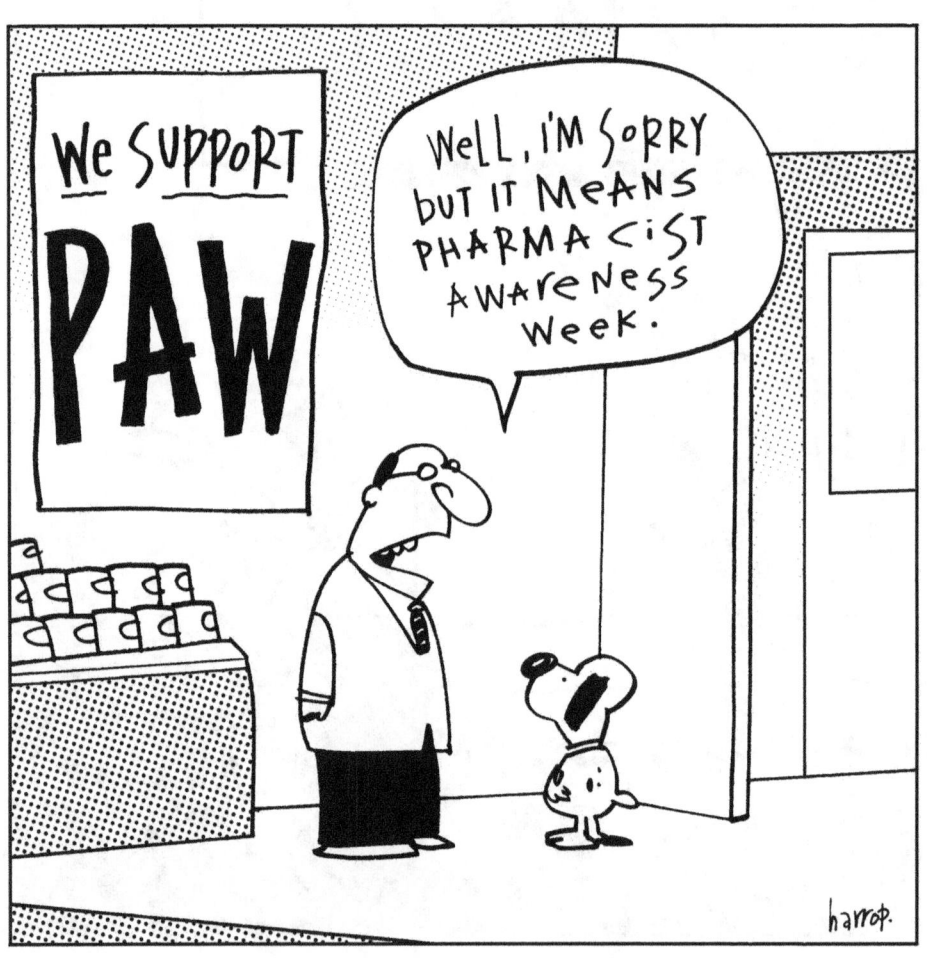

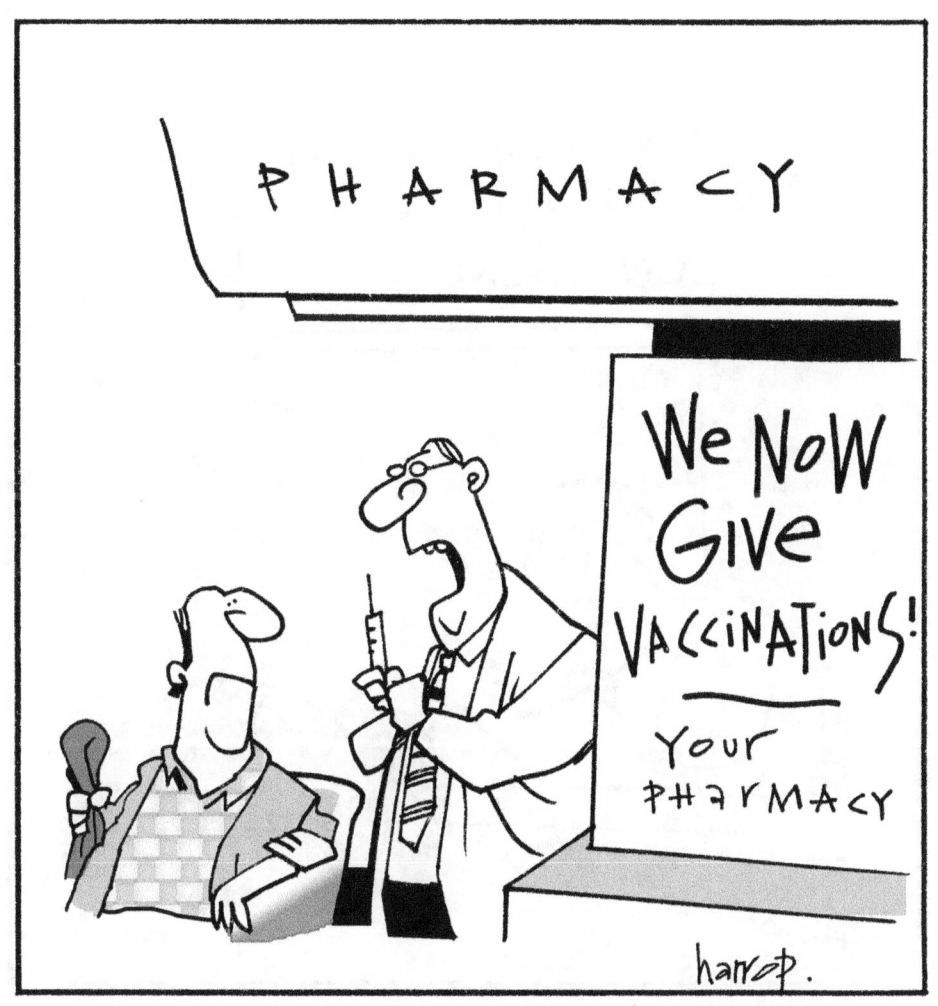

**Before I start ... remember needling ME
about my golf scores?**

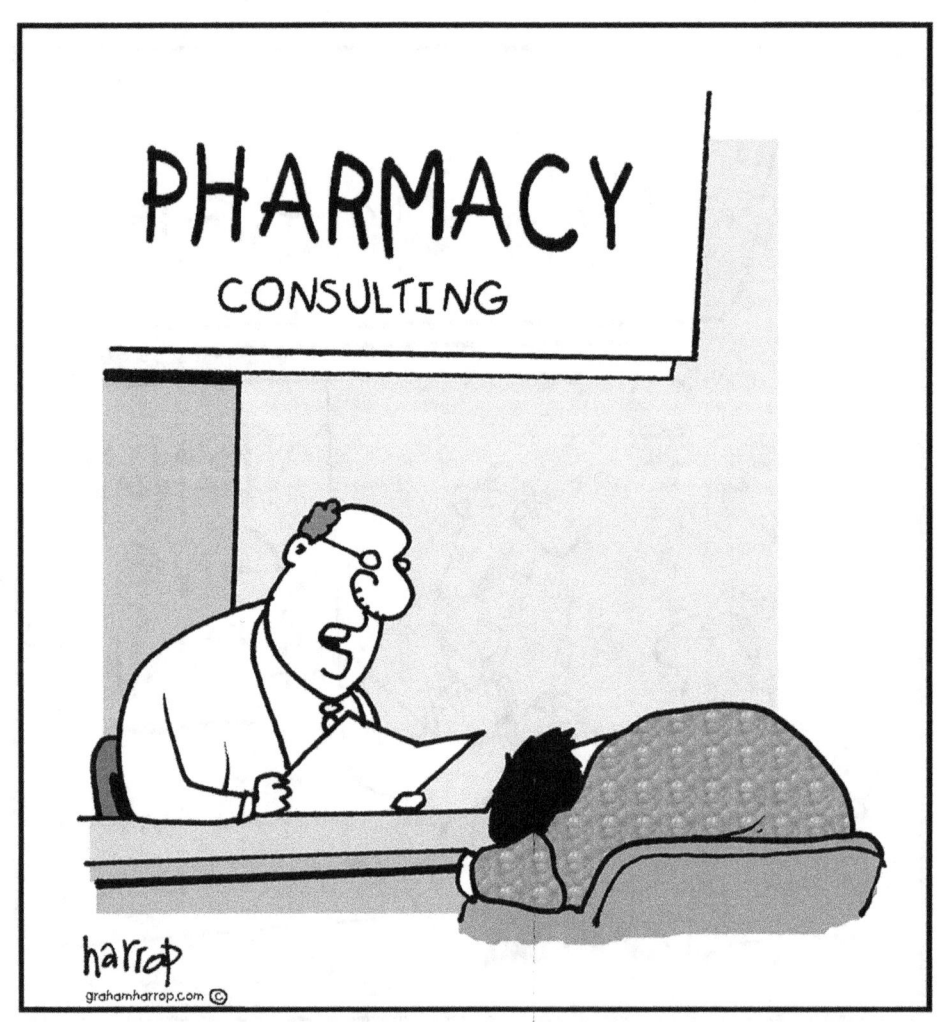

Frankly, I think you're overdoing it
on the sleep medication .

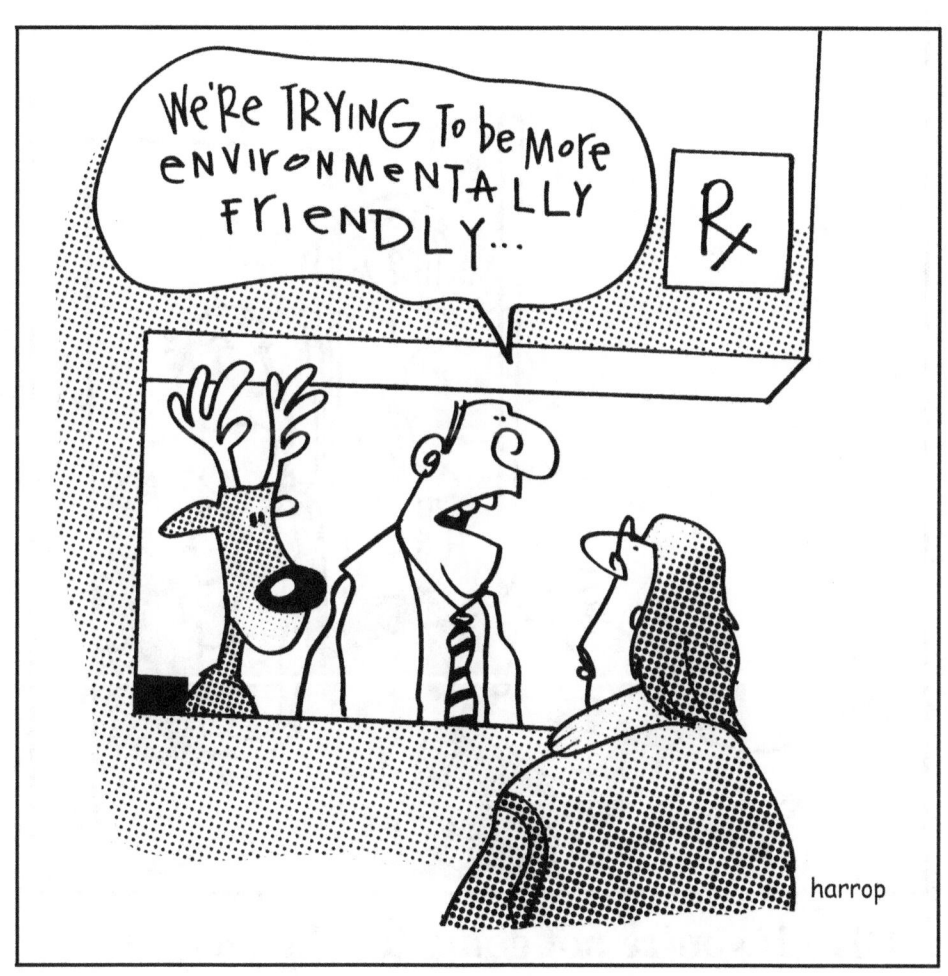

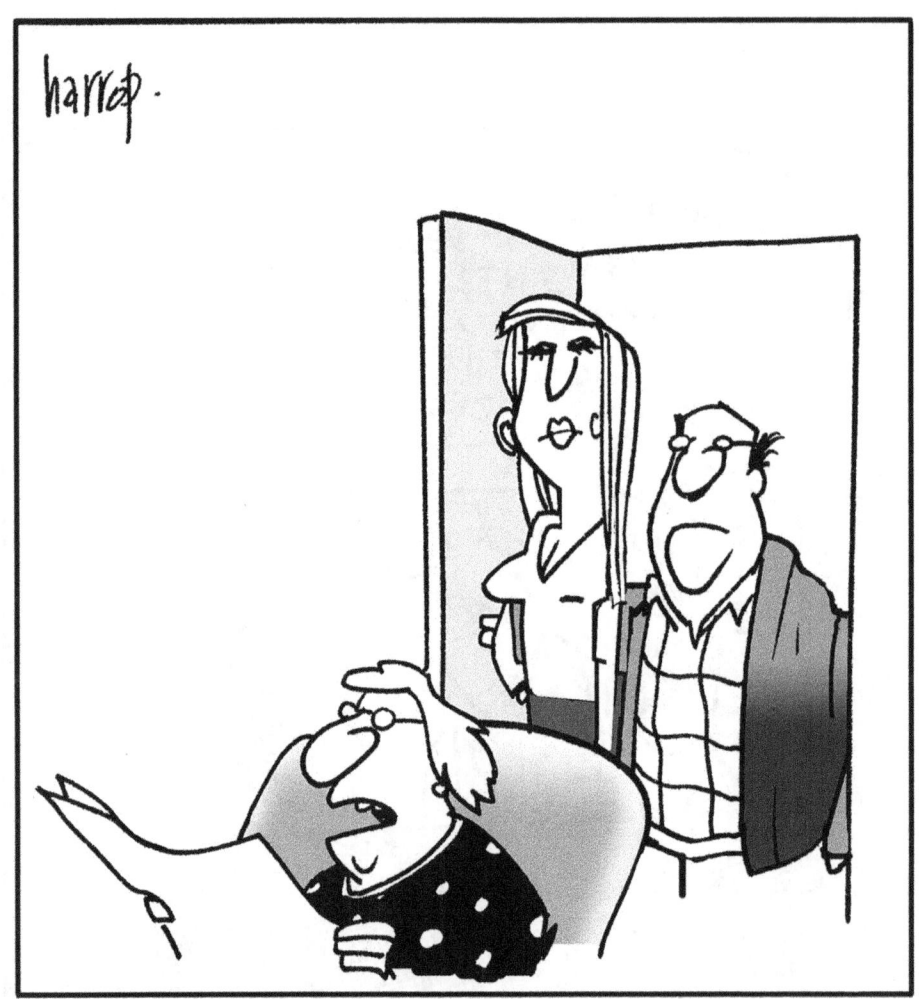

OK - if you're not going for the nicotine replacement therapies, how are you going to take your mind off cigarettes?

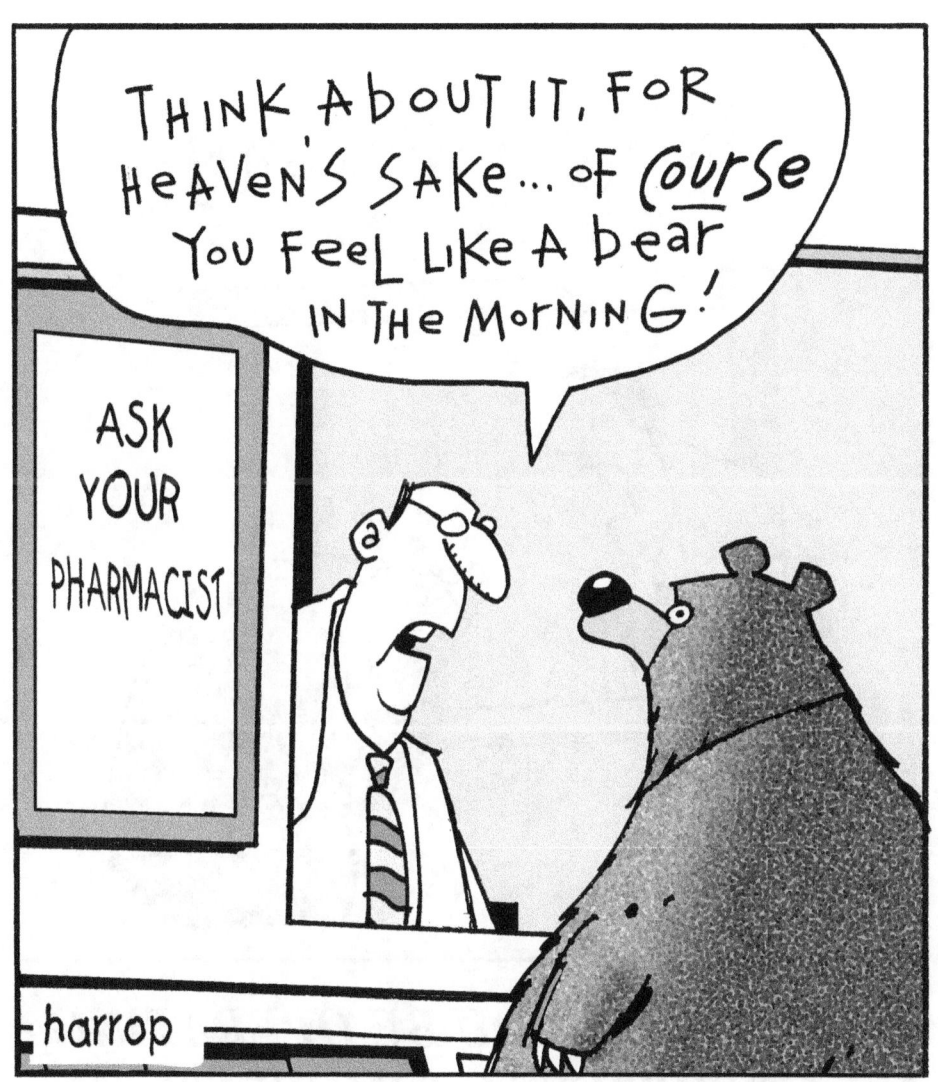

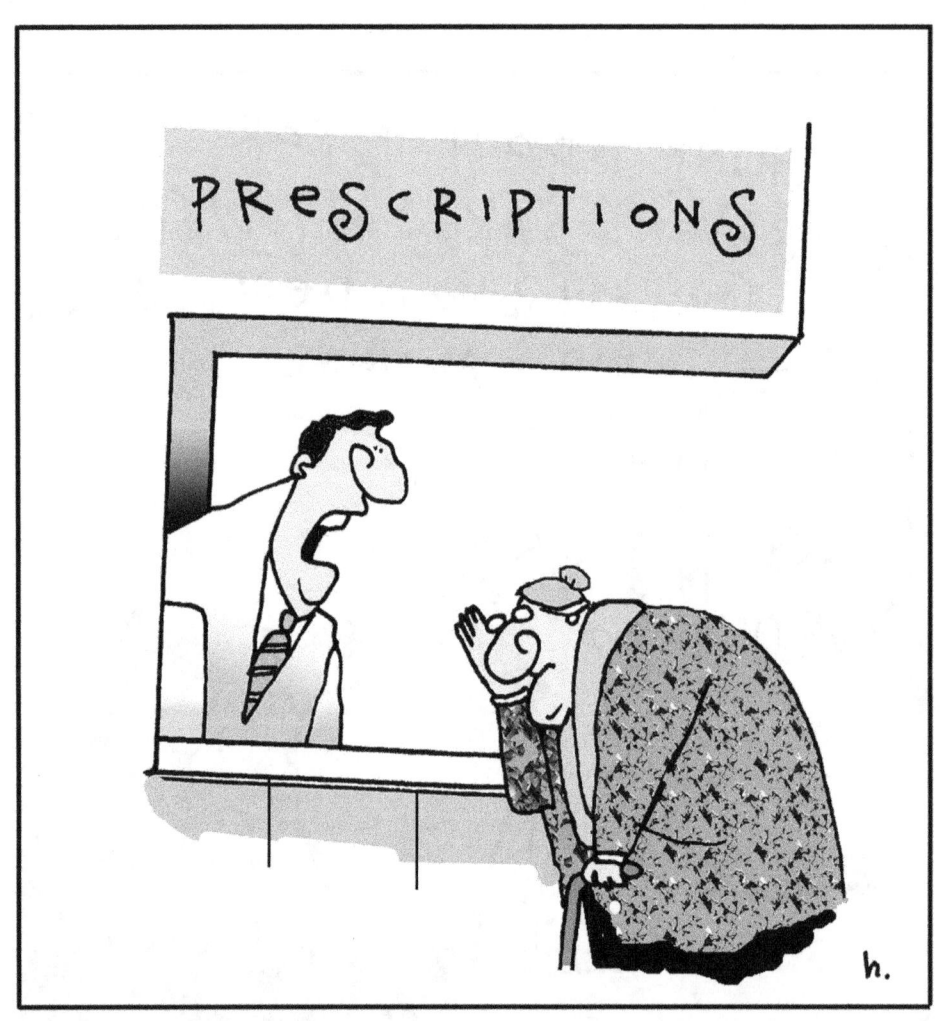

I SAID: 'WILL YOU BE OPERATING
ANY HEAVY MACHINERY?'

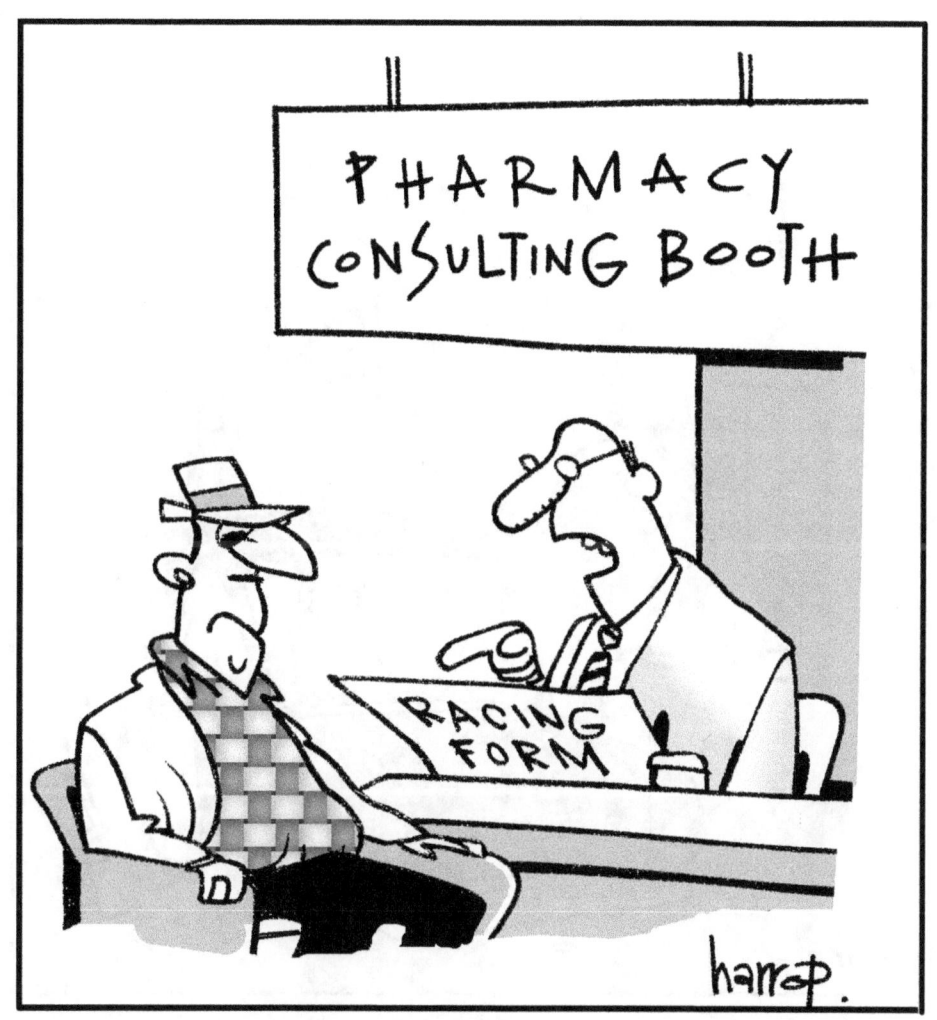

I usually just give advice on prescriptions,
but since you ask, I'm going to say:
'Dancing Boy' in the fourth!

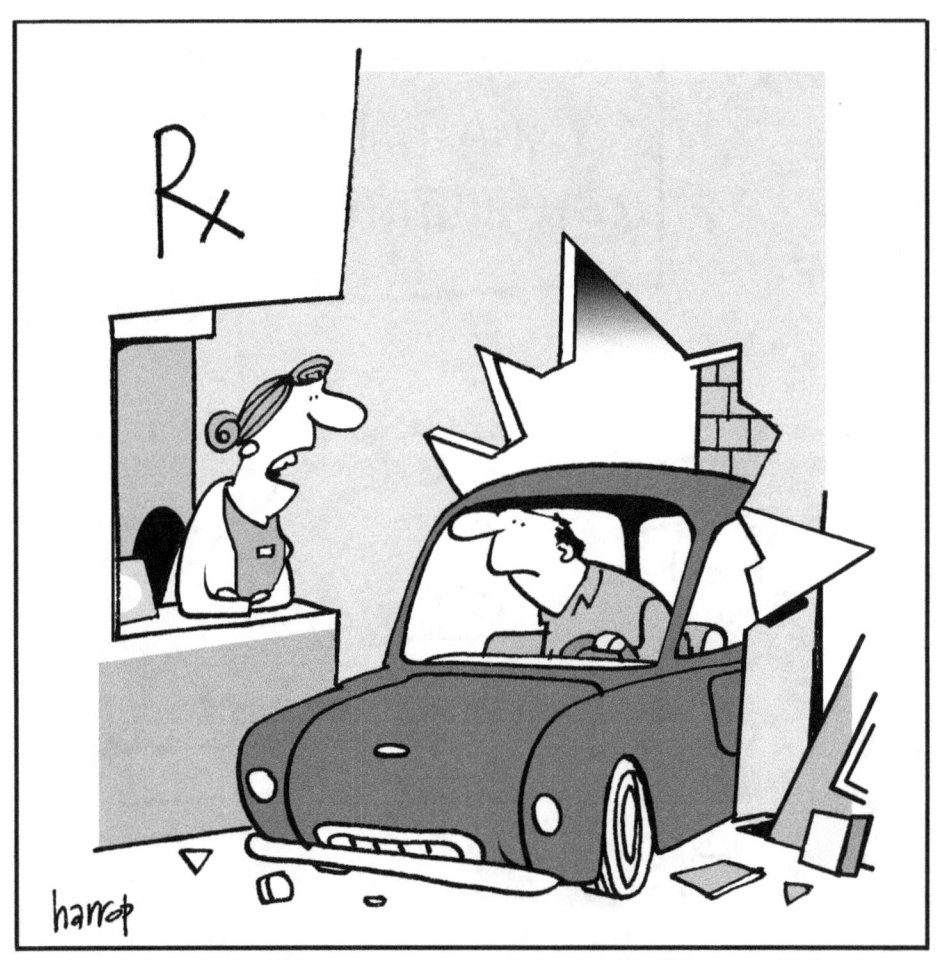

**Well, your friend was mistaken about this
being a drive-thru pharmacy!**

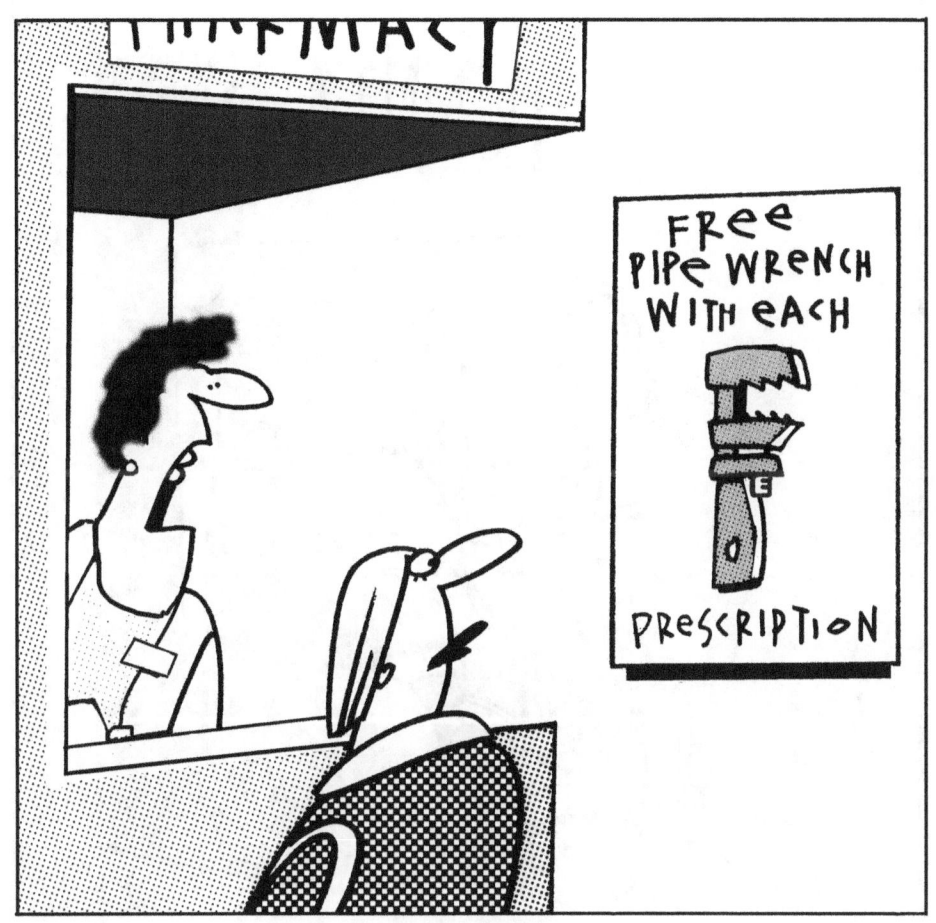

People are still having trouble opening the childproof safety caps...

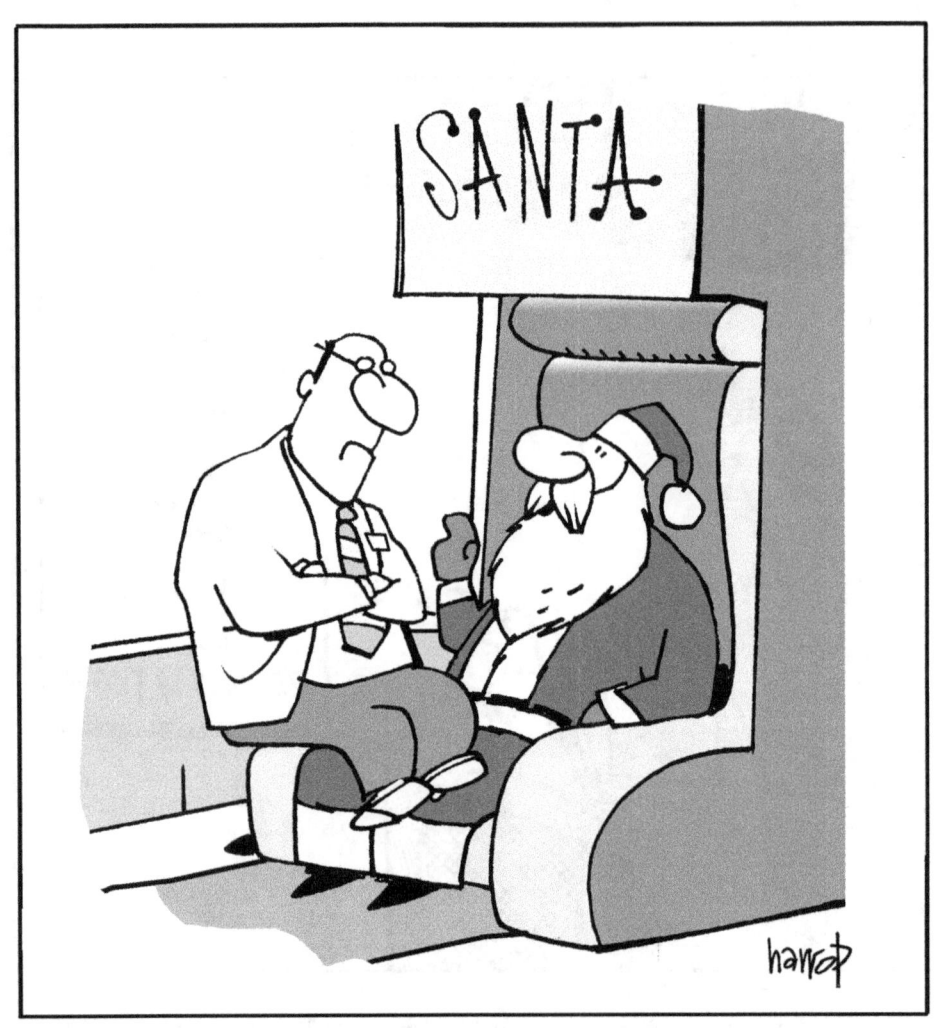

I told you *LAST* year - we don't make a 'L'il pharmacist' booblehead doll!

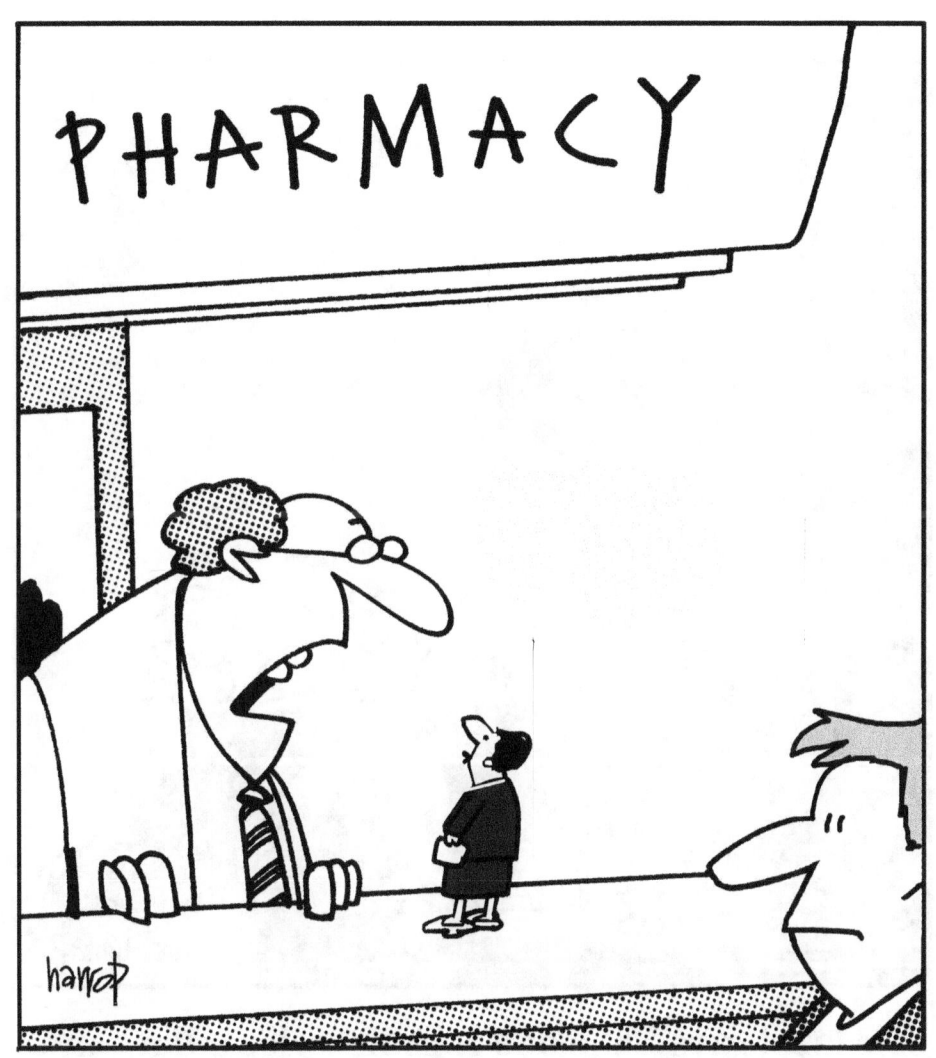

You're taking far too many diet pills ... !

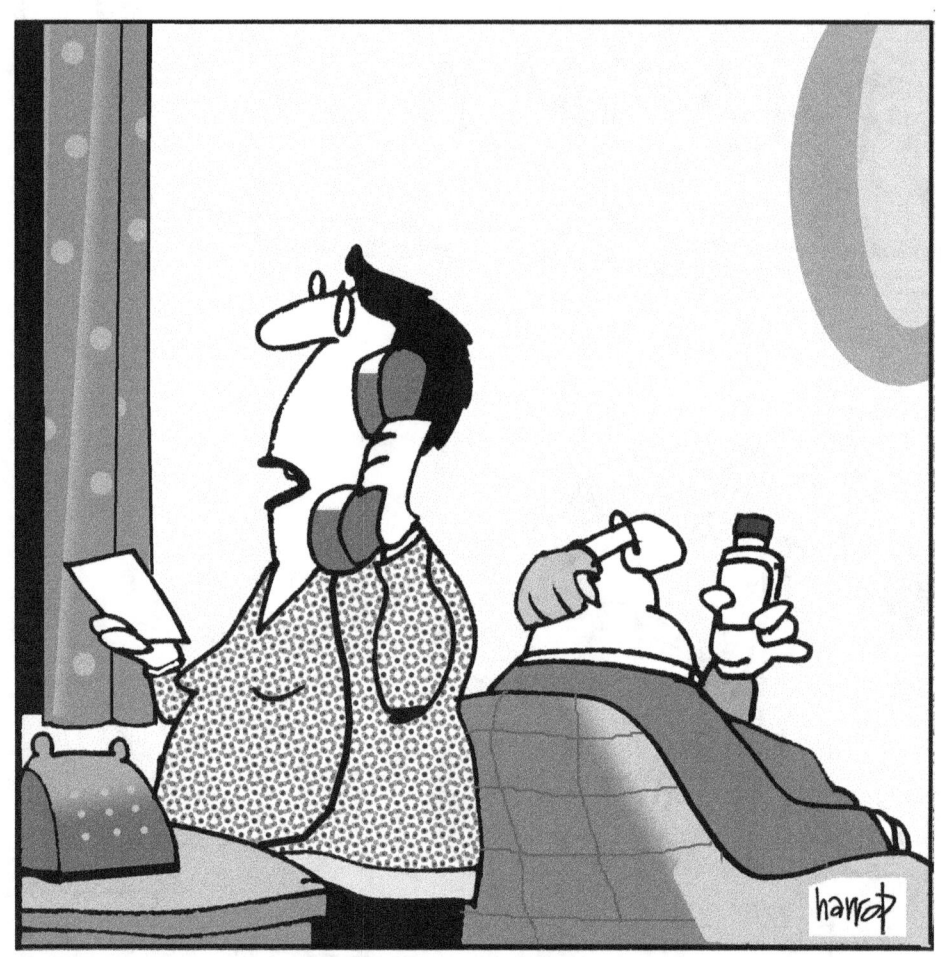

The label says 'take one capsule twice a day' and my husband wants to know which one...

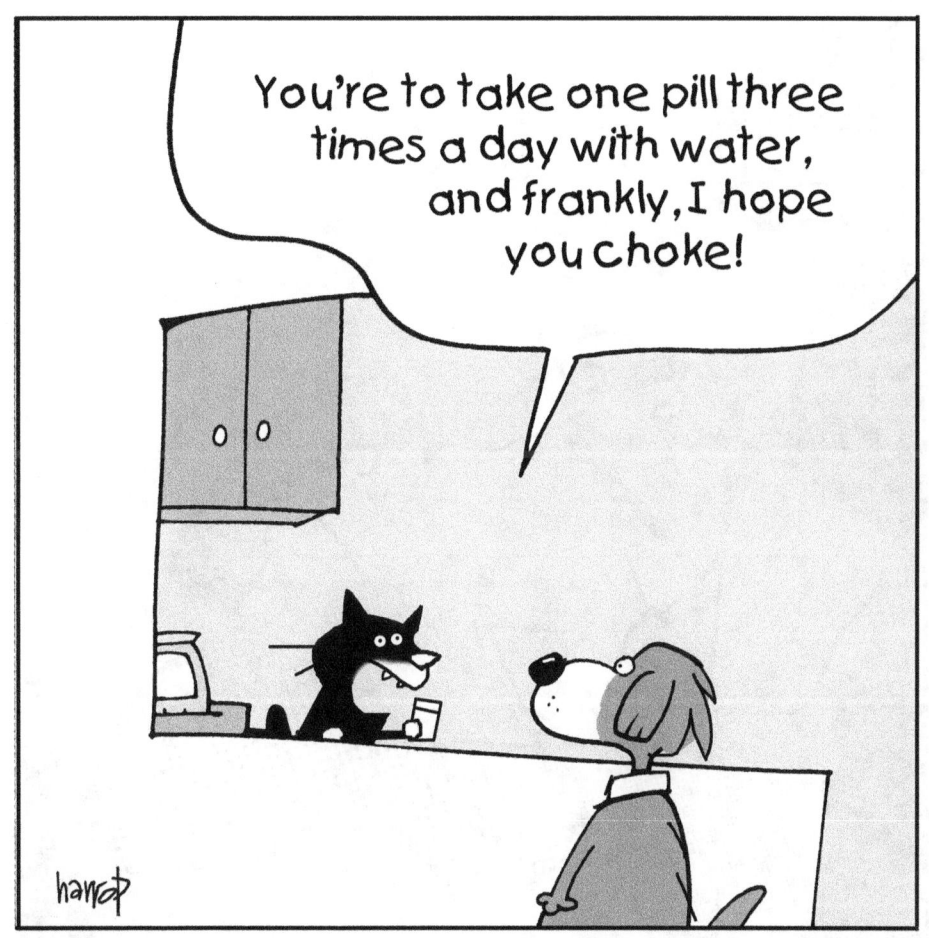

Why cats aren't allowed to run pharmacies

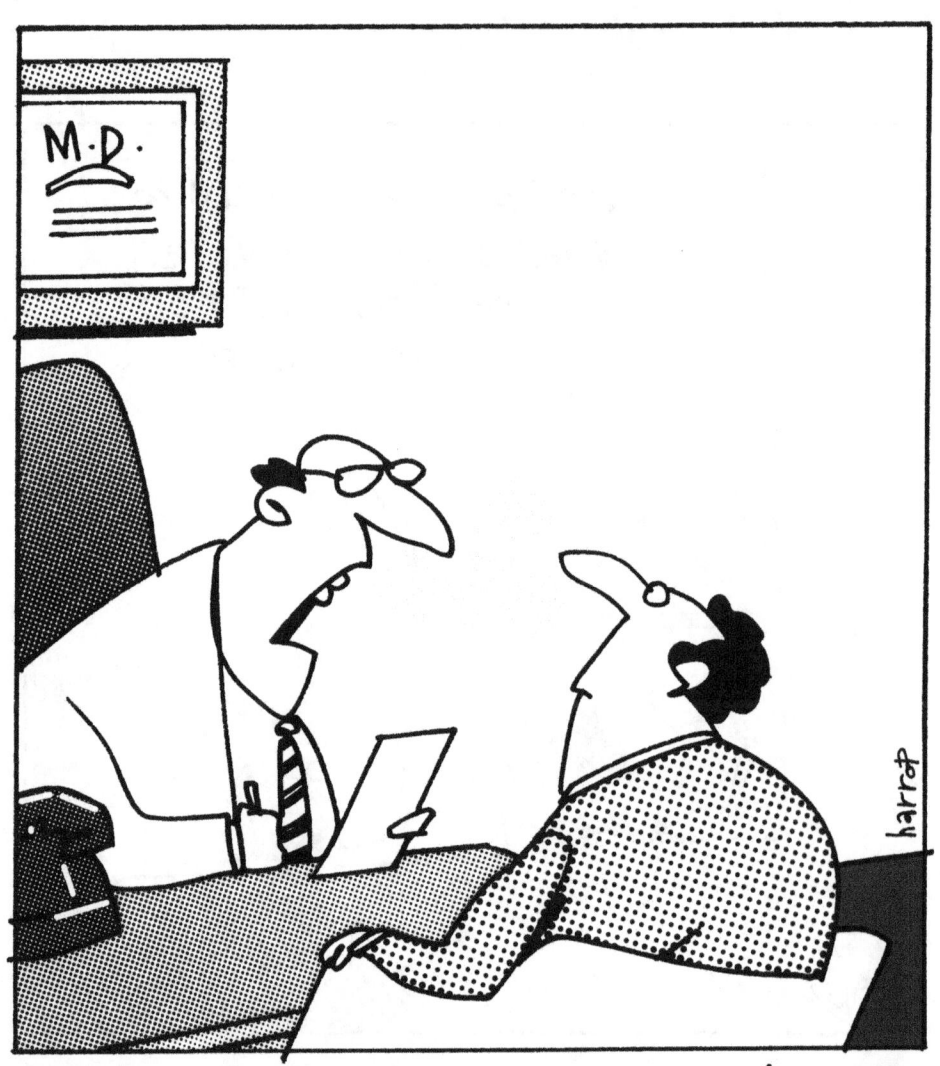

ONCE I TELL YOU HOW MUCH THE PILLS COST, I'M GOING TO HAVE TO ADD 'HIGH BLOOD PRESSURE' TO YOUR LIST OF AILMENTS.

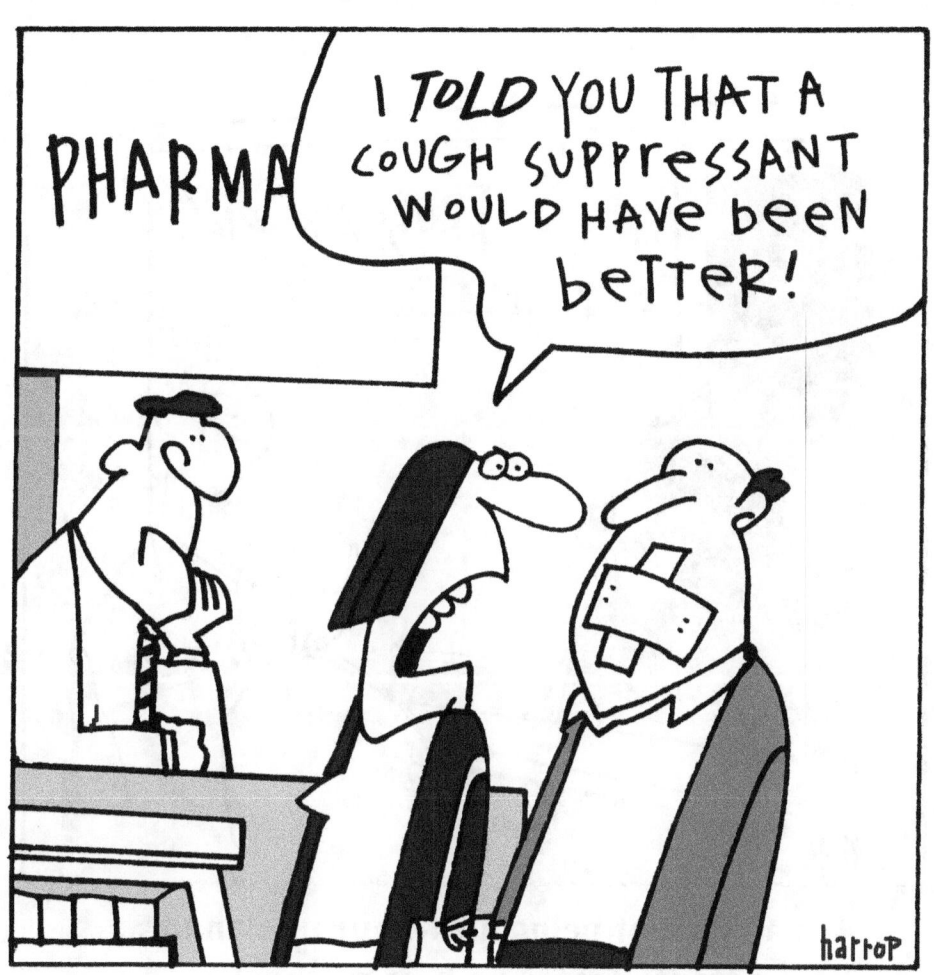

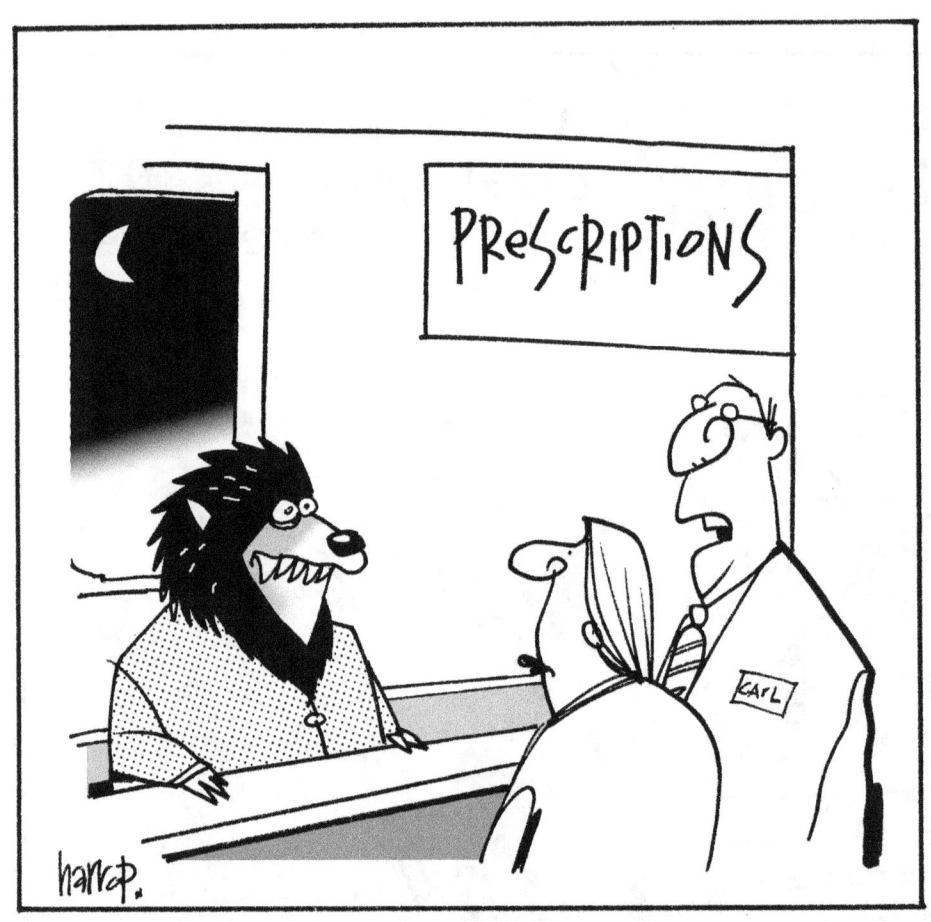

It's all part of being a 24-hour pharmacy...
he wants advice on hair removal.

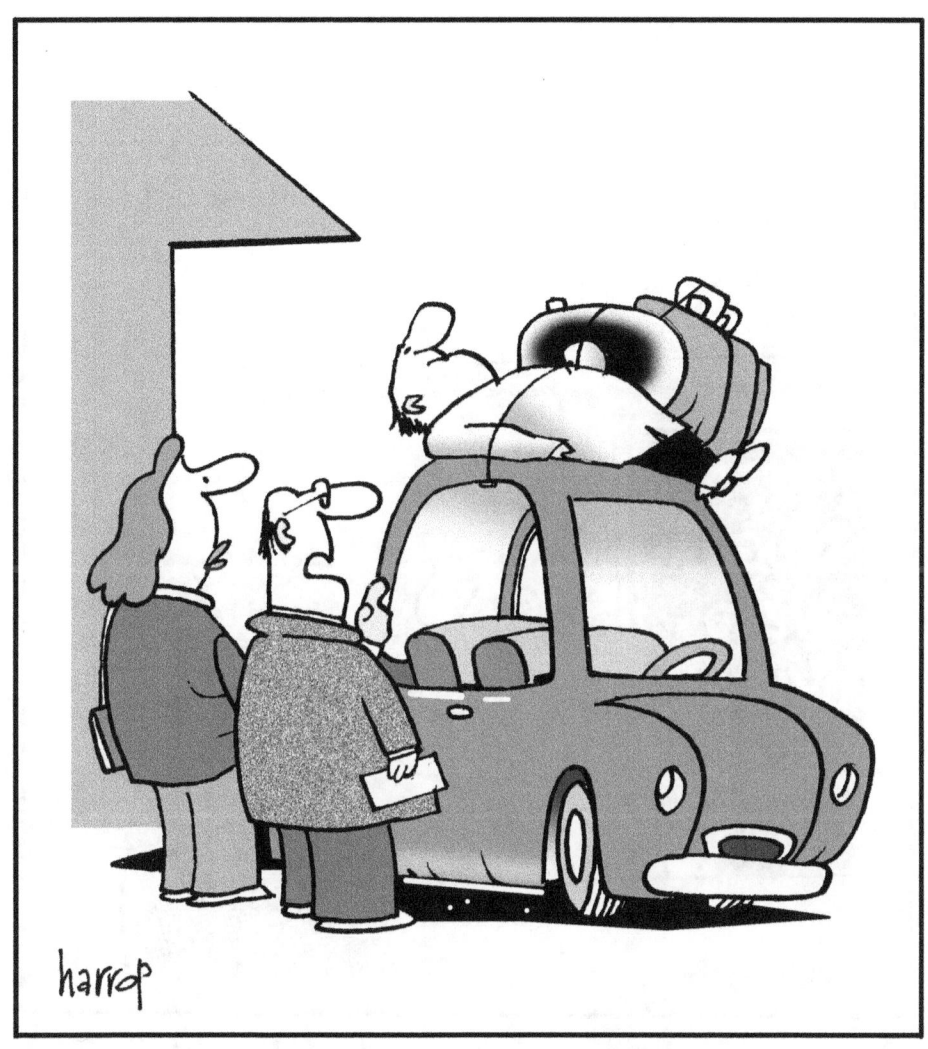

OK - have we got everything that we need for the trip? ... suitcases ... inner tube... friendly neighbourhood pharmacist...

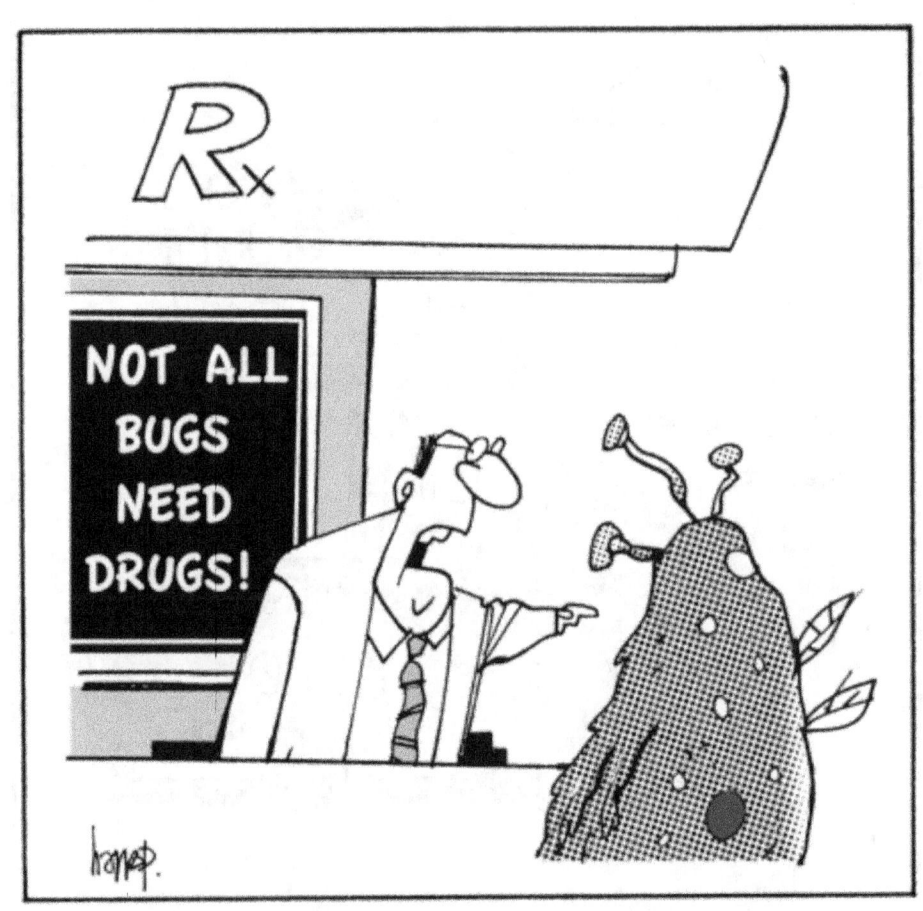

Look - I'm not prepared to debate it...
now *GET OUT!*

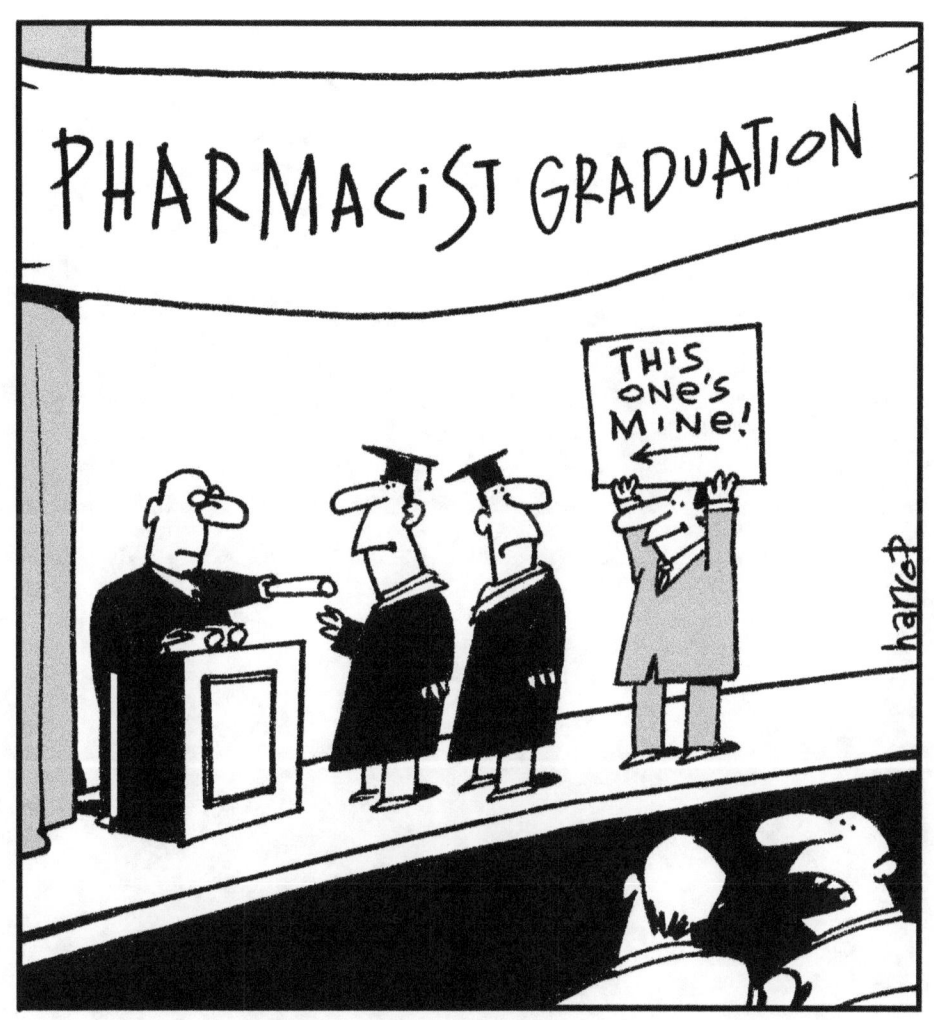

I think it has something to do with the
pharmacist shortage.

www.ingramcontent.com/pod-product-compliance
Lightning Source LLC
Chambersburg PA
CBHW080524190526
45169CB00008B/3049